Magic Mushrooms

A Practical Guide

copyrighted@2024

Joe Andre

Table of Contents

Chapter One

Introduction to Magic Mushrooms

Magic mushrooms, scientifically known as psilocybin mushrooms, have captured the human imagination for centuries with their mystical appeal and mind-altering properties. This chapter sets the stage for an exploration of the world of these mysterious fungi, delving into their origins, cultural significance and the legal environment that surrounds them.

1.1 What are magic mushrooms?

Magic mushrooms belong to the genus Psilocybe and other related genera that contain psychoactive compounds such as psilocybin and psilocin. These compounds interact with the human brain to induce altered states of consciousness, vivid hallucinations, and deep introspection. The effects are often described as a journey into the depths of the mind, unlocking the door to creativity, self-discovery and spiritual insight.

1.2 Historical perspectives

Magic mushrooms have been used historically from the dawn of humanity. Indigenous cultures around the world, from the Aztecs in Mesoamerica to shamans in

Siberia, have incorporated these mushrooms into their religious and medicinal practices. Their presence in religious ceremonies and rites of passage speaks to the profound impact they have had on human spirituality and cultural traditions.

1.3 Cultural Significance

The cultural significance of magic mushrooms transcends geographic boundaries. From traditional rituals to contemporary artistic expression, these mushrooms have left an indelible mark on human culture. Their influence extends to literature, art and music, with iconic figures such as Aldous Huxley and Terence McKenna advocating their exploration as tools for expanding consciousness.

1.4 Legal Status

Despite their rich history and cultural significance, the legal status of magic mushrooms varies worldwide. Some regions permit their use in religious or therapeutic contexts, while others strictly prohibit possession or cultivation. This section provides an overview of the current legal environment, emphasizing the importance of understanding and complying with local regulations.

Mushroom Kingdom

2.1 Anatomy and physiology of fungi

To understand the magic of magic mushrooms, we must delve into the complex anatomy and physiology that distinguishes mushrooms from other forms of life on Earth. From the tips of their hats to the depths of their mycelial networks, fungi weave a fascinating story of adaptation and interconnectedness.

2.1.1 The Mushroom Cap: A Crown of Mysteries

At the heart of every magic mushroom lies the hat, an

unmistakable feature that varies in color, shape and size from species to species. The cap serves as a protective shield for the gills below, protecting the delicate spore-producing structures from the elements. Looking at the mushroom hat is like peering into a miniature universe where spores await their journey into the unknown.

2.1.2 Gills: The Spore Factory

Beneath the cap, like the pages of a book, lies a labyrinthine network of gills that play a vital role in the mushroom's reproductive cycle. These gills contain countless microscopic cells, each with the potential to develop into spores. As the cap matures, the gills release spores into the air, starting the cycle of propagation and germination, thus sustaining the life of the fungus.

2.1.3 Stem: Support and guidance

The stem, often slender and strong, provides the cap with structural support and lifts it above the substrate. In addition to its role in structural integrity, the stem acts as a conduit to transport nutrients absorbed by the mycelium to the cap for spore production. Some mushrooms show a partial veil, a membrane that once covered the gills during early development and eventually detached when the cap expanded.

2.1.4 Mycelium: Underground network

Beneath the surface, hidden from view, the mycelium weaves an extensive network of filamentous structures. This network of mycelium serves as the true heart of the fungus, actively absorbing nutrients from the surrounding environment. Through a process known as hyphal growth, the mycelium examines and decomposes organic matter, which plays a key role in nutrient cycling and soil health.

2.2 Common types of magic mushrooms

Magic mushrooms belong to a diverse family of mushrooms, with each species having unique properties, appearance and psychoactive properties. Here we take a journey through the fascinating world of these mushrooms and explore some of the most famous and widely studied species.

2.2.1 Psilocybe cubensis: The Golden Teacher

Psilocybe cubensis is among the most widespread and well-known magic mushrooms. This species, characterized by its large golden-brown cap and distinctive veil, is known for its potency and distribution both in natural habitats and in cultivation. Psilocybe cubensis is often considered a "teacher" because of its potential for inducing deep insights and introspective experiences.

2.2.2 Psilocybe semilanceata: The Liberty Cap

Psilocybe semilanceata, named for its characteristic conical cap resembling a liberty cap, is found in various regions around the world. Its smaller size and subtle appearance make it a challenge to recognize, but its psychoactive properties are powerful. The Liberty Cap has a rich history, often associated with ancient European rituals and practices.

2.2.3 Psilocybe cyanescens: Wavy cap

Psilocybe cyanescens, recognized by its wavy or wavy cap, thrives in forests and grassy areas. This strain is known for its high levels of psilocybin and psilocin, which contribute to intense and vivid psychedelic experiences. The Wavy Cap has gained popularity among psychonauts and researchers alike for its unique properties.

2.2.4 Amanita muscaria: toadstool

Although not a true psilocybin-containing mushroom, Amanita muscaria deserves mention for its cultural significance and unique psychoactive compounds. Known for its iconic red cap adorned with white spots, the toadstool has been used in shamanic practices and folklore, producing effects distinct from psilocybin-containing mushrooms.

2.3 Growing Magic Mushrooms: A Beginner's Guide

Growing magic mushrooms is a transformative and enriching experience that allows enthusiasts to follow the entire life cycle of these mystical mushrooms. It provides a comprehensive beginner's guide that offers step-by-step instructions and insight into the art of growing magic mushrooms at home.

2.3.1 Getting started: Basic consumables

Before embarking on the magical journey of cultivation, collect the necessary supplies. This includes spore syringes, substrate (such as brown rice flour or vermiculite), glass containers, a pressure cooker, and a growing terrarium. The selection of high-quality spores and sterile equipment is crucial for successful cultivation.

2.3.2 Substrate preparation and inoculation

Create a nutrient-rich substrate by combining brown rice flour, vermiculite and water. Sterilize this mixture in glass containers using a pressure cooker to remove any competing microorganisms. After cooling, inoculate the substrate with spores from a syringe, ensuring an aseptic environment to avoid contamination.

2.3.3 Colonization and mycelial growth

Place the inoculated jars in a warm and dark environment for the mycelium to colonize the substrate. Mycelial growth appears as white, filamentous structures spreading throughout the substrate. Patience is key during this stage as it can take several weeks for the mycelium to fully colonize the substrate.

2.3.4 Birth and fertility

Once the substrate is fully colonized, transfer it to the terrarium for the fruiting stage. Maintain optimal conditions, including high humidity and fresh air exchange. The mushrooms will begin to emerge from the substrate, and over time the caps will expand, signaling their readiness for harvesting. The fetal phase usually lasts several weeks.

2.3.5 Harvesting and spore printing

Harvest mature mushrooms by gently twisting or cutting them

from the substrate. Collect spores for future cultivation by allowing mature caps to drop spores onto a sterile surface to create a spore imprint. This print can be used to inoculate new substrates and continue the culture cycle.

2.3.6 Tips and troubleshooting

To increase your growing success, pay attention to details such as keeping it clean, controlling environmental conditions, and lighting settings. Eliminate common problems such as contamination, stunted growth or abnormal development to ensure a bountiful harvest of powerful magic mushrooms.

Chapter Two

Psychedelic Compounds

3.1 Psilocybin and Psilocin: Magical Ingredients

At the heart of magic mushrooms lies a duo of enchanting compounds: psilocybin and its metabolite psilocin. These chemical entities are the alchemists behind the mystical experiences that occur when one partakes in the consumption of magic mushrooms.

3.1.1 Psilocybin: The Prophetic Prodrug

Psilocybin, a naturally occurring compound found in various

species of magic mushrooms, belongs to the tryptamine class. Notably, psilocybin itself is not psychoactive; rather, it serves as a prodrug; a precursor that is transformed into an active substance in the human body. This transformation is a key step on the alchemical journey from contention to transcendent experience.

3.1.2 Psilocin: Alchemical Elixir

After ingestion, psilocybin goes on a transformational journey in the human body. The liver plays the role of an alchemist, enzymatically converting psilocybin into its psychoactive form: psilocin. It is psilocin that dances with serotonin receptors in the brain and orchestrates the symphony of altered perception, vivid vision and deep introspection that characterizes the magic mushroom experience.

3.1.3 Tryptamine Harmony: Serotonin's Kin

Psilocybin and psilocin are structurally similar to serotonin, a neurotransmitter central to mood regulation. Their molecular similarity allows them to bind to serotonin receptors, especially the 5-HT2A receptor. This affinity leads to a cascade of events that alter neural activity and give rise to the kaleidoscopic mindscapes experienced during the psychedelic journey.

3.1.4 Dosage and effectiveness

The power of the magic mushroom experience is intricately linked to the concentration of psilocybin and psilocin in the mushrooms. Different species and even individual mushrooms can vary in their psychedelic content. Understanding dosage is critical to navigating the fine line between a gentle, introspective experience and a more intense, visually immersive journey.

3.2 How do magic mushrooms work?

The journey to magical realms induced by magic mushrooms is controlled by a complex dance of chemical compounds in the brain. Understanding how psilocybin and psilocin interact with the human neural landscape provides insight into the mechanics of the psychedelic experience.

3.2.1 Ingestion and metabolism

The journey begins with the ingestion of magic mushrooms, where psilocybin, the inactive prodrug, embarks on a transformative journey through the digestive system. The liver plays a key role in this alchemical process, converting psilocybin into its active form, psilocin. Once transformed, psilocin enters the center of the symphony of altered consciousness.

3.2.2 Affinity for the serotonin receptor

The magic of psilocin lies in its affinity for serotonin receptors, especially the 5-HT2A receptor. Serotonin, a neurotransmitter associated with mood regulation, shares structural similarities with psilocin. This similarity allows psilocin to bind to serotonin receptors and trigger a cascade of events that lead to a change in neural activity.

3.2.3 Neural connectivity and altered perception

The binding of psilocin to serotonin receptors results in a shift in neural connectivity, creating unusual patterns of communication between different areas of the brain. This altered connectivity is thought to underlie the profound changes in perception that occur during the magic mushroom journey. Time can stretch or compress, colors can intensify, and boundaries between self and environment can dissolve.

3.2.4 Network default mode and ego dissolution

Neuroimaging studies reveal that magic mushrooms induce changes in the default mode network (DMN), a network of brain regions associated with self-referential thoughts and the sense of ego. Psilocin appears to disrupt the normal functioning of the DMN, leading to the dissolution of ego boundaries. This dissolution of the ego is an essential aspect of the psychedelic experience, allowing individuals to transcend their habitual sense of self.

3.2.5 Variability of experience

The effects of magic mushrooms can vary greatly between individuals and even across different experiences for the same person. Factors such as dosage, setting and setting, and individual differences in brain chemistry contribute to this variability. The unpredictability of the psychedelic experience adds an element of mystery to every journey.

3.3 Science of altered states of consciousness

Magic mushrooms are more than just a collection of receptor-interacting molecules; they are gateways to altered states of consciousness. We will explore the scientific basis of how psilocybin and psilocin produce these profound shifts in consciousness and perception.

3.3.1 Neuroimaging Insights

Modern neuroscience has provided a window into brain activity during a psychedelic experience. Neuroimaging studies, including functional magnetic resonance imaging (fMRI) and positron emission tomography (PET), reveal altered patterns of neural connectivity. Areas that don't normally communicate with each other synchronize, giving rise to unique mental landscapes that you traverse during your journey to find magic mushrooms.

3.3.2 Default Mode Network (DMN) Disruption.

Central to the science of altered consciousness is the disruption of the default mode network (DMN). This network, associated with self-referential thoughts and the ego, undergoes changes in connectivity under the influence of psilocin. Dissolving the DMN contributes to a sense of ego dissolution where the boundaries between the self and the outside world become fluid.

3.3.3 Ego Dissolution and Mystical Experiences

Dissolution of the ego, a hallmark of the psychedelic experience, involves a temporary loss of one's sense of self. This phenomenon has been correlated with intense and mystical experiences. Studies suggest a link between the intensity of ego dissolution and reported positive outcomes, including increased well-being and a sense of interconnectedness.

3.3.4 Changed perception of time and space

Magic mushrooms have the power to disrupt the perception of time and space. Subjective experiences often involve a sense of time dilation or compression, where moments can seem eternal or pass in the blink of an eye. Spatial distortion contributes to the perception of vibrant colors, complex patterns and increased connection with the surrounding environment.

3.3.5 Therapeutic implications

The science of altered states of consciousness goes beyond research to potential therapeutic applications. Research suggests promising results in the treatment of a variety of mental health conditions, including depression, anxiety and PTSD. The ability of magic mushrooms to induce profound shifts in perspective may contribute to their therapeutic potential.

Chapter Three

Rituals and Traditions
4.1 Shamanic practices

Deeply rooted in ancient traditions, shamanic practices have used magical mushrooms as sacred tools for spiritual exploration, healing, and connection with the divine. This reveals the mystical realm of shamanism, where magical mushrooms are worshiped as keys to unlocking altered states of consciousness.

4.1.1 The shamanic path

Revered as spirit guides and healers in indigenous cultures, shamans embark on shamanic journeys facilitated by the visionary properties of magic mushrooms. These journeys often involve entering altered states of consciousness to communicate with spirits, gain insights, and obtain information beneficial to the individual or community.

4.1.2 Communication with spirits

Magical mushrooms are considered a medium for connection with the spirit world. In a shamanic context, the psychedelic experience is not a mere hallucination, but a sacred pathway where the shaman's consciousness transcends the mundane and enters realms inhabited by benevolent and malevolent spirits. Communicating with these entities serves a variety of purposes, including seeking guidance, healing, or divination.

4.1.3 Healing and Transformation

Shamans use the transformative power of magic mushrooms for healing purposes. The altered states induced by these mushrooms are believed to facilitate the identification and resolution of spiritual, emotional or physical ailments. Through the shamanic journey, individuals can undergo profound transformations, emerging with newfound insights, balance, and a renewed connection to the spiritual fabric of existence.

4.1.4 Rituals and Ceremonies

Shamanic rituals with magic mushrooms are carefully structured events. They often involve ceremonial practices such as chanting, drumming, and ritual dancing to induce a trance-like state. The environment is carefully chosen to create a sacred space and heighten the individual's receptivity to the mystical experiences that magic mushrooms make possible.

4.1.5 Integration and sharing of wisdom

The shamanic journey is not considered complete with the end of the psychedelic experience. Integration is a crucial aspect where the wisdom gained from the journey is incorporated into everyday life. Shamans can share their knowledge with the community and act as mediators of healing and wisdom.

4.2 Indigenous use of magic mushrooms

Magic mushrooms are an integral part of the spiritual and cultural practices of indigenous communities around the world. This illuminates the rich tapestry of traditions, beliefs and ceremonies surrounding the use of magic mushrooms in various indigenous cultures.

4.2.1 Mazatec tradition in Mexico

In Mexico, the Mazatecs have a long history of using magic mushrooms, especially Psilocybe cubensis, in their spiritual rituals. Under the guidance of wise healers known as curanderos or curanderas, individuals participate in sacred ceremonies in which mushrooms are ingested to facilitate connection with the divine, receive guidance, and promote healing. Mazatec tradition emphasizes respect for mushrooms and the spirits they invoke.

4.2.2 The original inhabitants of Central and South America

In addition to Mexico, various indigenous groups in Central and South America have incorporated magical mushrooms into their cosmologies and ceremonies. In Amazonian regions, mushrooms such as Psilocybe cubensis are used along with other herbal medicines during ayahuasca ceremonies. These rituals are central to the cultural identity of indigenous tribes and foster a deep connection to nature, ancestors and the spiritual realm.

4.2.3 Amanita muscaria in Siberian shamanism

In Siberian shamanism, Amanita muscaria, commonly known as toadstool, plays an important role in rituals. Siberian shamans consume this striking red-capped mushroom to induce altered states of consciousness. Amanita muscaria's distinctive appearance with its red cap and white spots has led to its symbolic association with spiritual realms and magical paths.

4.2.4 Connection with nature and ancestors

The indigenous use of magic mushrooms is deeply connected to a respect for nature and a belief in interconnectedness. These mushrooms are not only consumed for personal insight, but are seen as channels for communication with the natural world, ancestral spirits, and unseen forces that shape the fabric of existence.

4.2.5 Preserving traditions

Despite external pressures and cultural shifts, some indigenous communities are trying to preserve their sacred traditions involving magic mushrooms. Efforts are being made to pass down the knowledge from one generation to the next, ensuring that the spiritual significance of these mushrooms remains an integral part of their cultural heritage.

4.3 Modern rituals and ceremonies

Nowadays, a resurgence of interest in magic mushrooms has given rise to modern rituals and ceremonies. This explores a deliberate and structured environment where individuals engage with magic mushrooms, drawing inspiration from traditional practices while adapting to the needs of the present.

4.3.1 Psychedelic ceremonies and facilitators

Modern psychedelic ceremonies often take place in carefully prepared settings with skilled facilitators guiding participants on their journeys. Drawing on insights from shamanic traditions and psychological frameworks, these facilitators aim to create a safe and supportive environment for individuals to explore the depths of their consciousness. To increase the therapeutic and transformative potential of the experience, there is an emphasis on setting and setting, setting intention, and communal support.

4.3.2 Integration circles

Integration circles after the ceremony have become an integral part of modern rituals. Participants come together to share their experiences, insights and challenges in a supportive group environment. These discussions are led by facilitators who help individuals integrate the lessons learned during the psychedelic experience into their daily lives. Integration circles contribute to a continuous process of personal growth and self-discovery.

4.3.3 Careful consumption

Modern magic mushroom rituals often involve a mindful approach to consumption. Participants are encouraged to approach the experience with intention, cultivate a sense of reverence for the mushrooms, and recognize the potential for personal transformation. Mindful consumption emphasizes the importance of individual responsibility and respect for the powerful nature of the psychedelic journey.

4.3.4 Music and artistic expression

Sound and artistic elements are often incorporated into modern rituals to enhance the overall experience. Known for its ability to influence mood and perception, music is carefully selected to complement the journey. Artistic expression, including visual art and movement, allows individuals to externalize and explore the inner landscapes encountered during the psychedelic experience.

4.3.5 Legal and Ethical Considerations

In regions where the legal environment allows, modern rituals operate within legal frameworks and ensure the safety and well-being of participants. Ethical considerations such as informed consent, responsible use, and commitment to harm minimization guide the facilitators and organizers of these ceremonies.

Chapter Four

Personal Experience
5.1 Tripping Safely: Set and setting

Embarking on a journey with magic mushrooms requires careful consideration of the environment and mindset, collectively referred to as "set and setting". This explores the importance of creating a conducive environment and setting for a safe and positive psychedelic experience.

5.1.1 Meaning of set and setting

The set and setting, often created by Timothy Leary, encapsulate the psychological and physical context in which the psychedelic experience takes place. The hunting ability (attitude) of the individual and the environment (attitude) greatly influence the nature and outcome of the trip. Creating a deliberate and comfortable setup and setup is paramount to a positive experience.

5.1.2 Mindset (set): intention and mental state

The mindset or state of mind of the individual plays a key role in shaping the psychedelic experience. Setting clear intentions before a trip allows individuals to focus on specific aspects of their lives, such as personal growth, self-discovery, or emotional healing. Cultivating a positive and open mind makes for a rewarding experience.

5.1.3 Environment (setting): Safe and comfortable spaces

The physical environment where the psychedelic experience takes place is the setting. Creating a safe, comfortable and familiar space minimizes external stressors and contributes to a sense of security. Factors such as lighting, music and the presence of trusted individuals can greatly influence the overall atmosphere.

5.1.4 Nature and exterior settings

For many, nature is the ideal environment for journeys in search of magical mushrooms. The tranquility of natural environments, such as forests, meadows or beaches, enhances the connection with the environment and heightens the sense of wonder. The outdoor environment also offers a spacious and free-spirited atmosphere for exploration.

5.1.5 Minimization of interference

A quiet and controlled environment helps minimize distractions during the trip.

Turning off your phones, creating a playlist of soothing music, and informing others around you of your journey makes for a focused and immersive experience. Distractions can disrupt the flow of introspection and hinder the potential therapeutic benefits of the journey.

5.1.6 Role of Trip Sitters

In certain situations, a trusted and experienced security guard can feel safe. A lifeguard provides reassurance, guidance and assistance in case of problems. This should be someone who is familiar with the effects of psychedelics and is able to offer support without imposing their own experiences on the individual.

5.2 Exploring the Inner Realms

Revered for their ability to unlock inner realms of consciousness, magical mushrooms invite individuals to embark on deep journeys within themselves. Here we delve into the introspective and transformative aspects of magic mushroom experiences and explore the realms of the mind that these mushrooms reveal.

5.2.1 Introspection and self-discovery

Magic mushrooms have a unique ability to catalyze introspection and invite the individual to explore the depths of their mind. Participants often encounter repressed emotions, unresolved trauma, and aspects of their personality that may be hidden from conscious awareness. This process of self-discovery contributes to personal growth and emotional healing.

5.2.2 Emotional release and catharsis

A psychedelic experience can act as a catalyst for emotional release and catharsis. Participants may find themselves expressing and processing deep-seated emotions, leading to a profound sense of relief and liberation. This emotional cleansing is often considered a therapeutic aspect of the magic mushroom journey.

5.2.3 Symbolic representation and archetypes

The inner realms explored during a magic mushroom experience are often rich in symbolic imagery and archetypal themes. Participants can encounter vivid visuals and symbols that have personal meaning or resonate with universal themes. These symbols can serve as gateways to

deeper layers of the
subconscious.

5.2.4 Transcending Time and Ego

Magic mushrooms have the power to dissolve the conventional sense of time and ego. Participants can experience a timeless quality during the journey, where past, present and future converge in a unique moment. Dissolving the boundaries of the ego can lead to a deep sense of interconnectedness with the universe and a transcendent understanding of one's place in the cosmic tapestry.

5.2.5 Spiritual Insights and Transcendence

Many individuals report experiencing spiritual insights and moments of transcendence during their magic mushroom journeys. These insights can include a sense of oneness with all living beings, a connection to higher states of consciousness, and a deep understanding of the interconnected nature of existence. These mystical aspects add to the spiritual dimensions of the psychedelic experience.

5.2.6 Integration and Application

The knowledge gained from exploring the inner realms during the magic mushroom experience is an integral part of the integration process. Participants engage in reflections, journals, and discussions to incorporate these experiences into their daily lives. The lessons learned contribute to permanent personal growth and a deeper understanding of oneself.

5.3 Integration of psychedelic experiences

The magic mushroom journey is not limited to the duration of the psychedelic experience; extends to the period after the journey.

Here we explore the key process of integration, where individuals weave the insights gained along the journey into the fabric of their daily lives.

5.3.1 Meaning of integration

Integration is a deliberate process of incorporating insights and experiences from psychedelic journeys into one's own life. It bridges the gap between the extraordinary realms visited during the magic mushroom experience and the practical everyday reality of existence. Integration is a critical component to maximizing the therapeutic benefits and long-term impact of psychedelic experiences.

5.3.2 Reflection and Journaling

Reflection plays a central role in the integration process. Participants often engage in journaling to capture the nuances of their experiences, emotions, and insights. Translating the unspeakable into written words helps to consolidate the knowledge gained and provides a reference point for future reflections.

5.3.3 Integration circles and community support

Integration circles, group discussions or therapy sessions offer a common space for individuals to share their experiences and insights. This shared exploration provides support, validation, and different perspectives, enhancing the collective understanding of the psychedelic journey. Community support fosters a sense of connection and shared growth.

5.3.4 Creative expression and art

Artistic expression becomes a powerful tool for integrating psychedelic experiences. Through various forms of creative expression, such as visual art, music, dance, or writing, individuals externalize the inner landscapes they encounter along the way. This process allows for a deeper exploration and communication of symbolic images and insights.

5.3.5 Mindfulness and meditation

Mindfulness and meditation practices serve as anchors for integrating psychedelic experiences. Cultivating a daily routine of mindfulness allows individuals to stay connected to the insights gained along the way. It promotes increased awareness of the present moment and promotes a sense of inner peace and clarity.

5.3.6 Lifestyle changes and personal growth

Integration often involves making conscious lifestyle changes based on the insights gained. Individuals can try to align their lives more closely with their values, prioritize self-care, and cultivate positive habits. These intentional changes contribute to permanent personal growth and the embodiment of the acquired experience.

5.3.7 Support for professional integration

In some cases, it may be beneficial to seek professional integration support. Psychedelic integration therapists or counselors provide guidance, tools, and a structured framework for individuals going through the integration process. This therapeutic support helps individuals solve problems, increase self-awareness, and promote ongoing growth.

Chapter Five

Health and Safety

6.1 Potential benefits of magic mushrooms

Research on magic mushrooms goes beyond their mystical and hallucinogenic properties. This study examines the potential therapeutic benefits associated with the use of magic mushrooms, drawing on a growing body of research and anecdotal evidence.

6.1.1 Alleviation of depression and anxiety

Research suggests that magic mushrooms, especially psilocybin, may have antidepressant and anxiolytic effects. Studies have shown that a single dose of psilocybin in a controlled and supportive environment can lead to a significant reduction in symptoms of depression and anxiety in individuals with treatment-resistant illnesses.

6.1.2 Improving emotional well-being

Magic mushrooms have been associated with improving emotional well-being and mood. Individuals often report an increased sense of gratitude, interconnectedness, and an overall positive shift in their emotional states after a psychedelic experience.

6.1.3 Facilitating psychotherapeutic processes

Psychotherapeutic applications of magic mushrooms are gaining recognition. Led by trained therapists, psilocybin therapy has shown promise in addressing a variety of mental health conditions, including post-traumatic stress disorder (PTSD), addiction, and existential distress in individuals facing life-threatening illnesses.

6.1.4 Encouraging creativity and problem solving

Magic mushrooms can have cognitive effects that increase creativity and problem solving. Users often report an increased capacity for divergent thinking, greater insight and a new perspective on long-term challenges. These cognitive benefits go beyond the acute psychedelic experience.

6.1.5 Spiritual and existential insights

Magic mushrooms are known to induce deep spiritual and existential experiences. These experiences can contribute to greater meaning, connectedness, and re-evaluation of one's place in the universe. For some individuals, these insights have a lasting impact on their spiritual and existential beliefs.

6.1.6 Smoking cessation and addiction treatment

Preliminary research suggests that magic mushrooms may have potential in the treatment of addictions, including nicotine addiction. Psilocybin-assisted therapy has shown promise in aiding smoking cessation, with participants reporting decreased appetite and increased likelihood of abstinence.

6.1.7 Palliative care and end-of-life anxiety

Magic mushrooms have been investigated as an adjunctive therapy in the palliative care setting. Psilocybin-assisted therapy has been shown to be effective in reducing anxiety at the end of life and provides a sense of peace and acceptance to individuals facing terminal illness.

6.1.8 Neuroplasticity and neural repair

New research shows that psychedelics, including magic mushrooms, can affect neuroplasticity and promote neural repair. This has implications for conditions involving neurodegeneration, although further research is needed to fully understand the mechanisms and potential applications.

6.2 Risks and side effects

While magic mushrooms have therapeutic potential, it is essential to be aware and understand the potential risks and side effects associated with their use. This explores the darker aspects of the magic mushroom experience and highlights the importance of informed and responsible engagement.

6.2.1 Challenging experiences

Journeys for magic mushrooms can sometimes lead to challenging or difficult experiences. Intense emotions, anxiety and feelings of paranoia may occur. Navigating these challenging states requires a supportive environment, a positive mindset, and in certain cases, the assistance of a trusted sitter.

6.2.2 Risk of psychosis

Individuals predisposed to psychotic disorders may be at

increased risk of experiencing psychotic-like symptoms during their magic mushroom journey. It is crucial for individuals with a personal or family history of psychosis to approach these substances with caution and under the guidance of a mental health professional.

6.2.3 HPPD (persistent hallucinogenic perception disorder)

Hallucinogen Persistent Perceptual Disorder, or HPPD, is a rare but documented phenomenon where individuals experience persistent visual disturbances or hallucinations long after the psychedelic trip has ended. The exact cause of HPPD is not fully understood, and research into the condition continues.

6.2.4 Flashbacks and intrusive thoughts

Some individuals may experience flashbacks or intrusive thoughts related to their psychedelic experiences. These moments might cause distress and interfere with day-to-day activities. Individuals struggling with persistent anxious thoughts should seek support from mental health professionals.

6.2.5 Impaired judgment and safety concerns

The altered state of consciousness induced by magic mushrooms can impair judgment and coordination. Engaging in activities that require fine motor skills such as driving, operating machinery, or crossing busy streets poses a safety risk and is strongly discouraged during the psychedelic experience.

6.2.6 Interactions with certain drugs

Magic mushrooms, specifically the psychedelic compounds psilocybin and psilocin, can interact with various medications. Combining these substances with drugs such as SSRIs, MAOIs or other psychiatric drugs can lead to adverse reactions. It is essential to consult a healthcare professional before using magic mushrooms, especially for individuals taking prescription medications.

6.2.7 Legal Consequences

The legal status of magic mushrooms varies globally and even within certain jurisdictions. Possession, cultivation and distribution of magic mushrooms can have legal consequences. Individuals should know and follow the laws governing these substances in their respective localities.

6.2.8 Physical discomfort and nausea

Magic mushrooms can cause physical discomfort, including nausea, vomiting, and stomach cramps. These side effects are more common during the early stages of the journey and are often referred to as "onset". Some individuals may find these sensations uncomfortable and should be prepared to handle potential physical discomfort.

6.3 Responsible use and damage reduction

Responsible use and harm reduction are fundamental principles for individuals dealing with magic mushrooms. This explores practical guidelines and strategies aimed at minimizing risk, promoting well-being and promoting a safe and informed approach to the use of these mushrooms.

6.3.1 Education and informed decision making

Education is the cornerstone of responsible use. Individuals considering mushroom use should thoroughly educate themselves about the effects, potential risks, and legal status of these substances. Informed decision-making enables individuals to navigate experiences responsibly.

6.3.2 Dosing and Gradual Escalation

Dosage plays a vital role in the nature and intensity of the magic mushroom experience. Starting with a low dose and gradually escalating, commonly known as "start low, go slow," allows individuals to acclimate to the effects and gauge their sensitivity. Understanding the potency of a specific type of mushroom is essential for responsible dosing.

6.3.3 Set and Setting Considerations

Creating a favorable file and setup is essential for a positive experience. Choosing a comfortable, familiar, and safe environment, along with adopting a positive and open mindset, increases the likelihood of a positive experience while minimizing the risk of anxiety or challenging episodes.

6.3.4 Trip Sitters and Support System

Having a trusted and experienced ranger can provide valuable support during your magic mushroom journey. The trip should be someone familiar with the effects of psychedelics, able to offer reassurance and ready to help in case of problems. Mutual trust and open communication are crucial.

6.3.5 Mindfulness and Intention Setting

Approaching the experience with mindfulness and setting clear intentions contributes to a positive and meaningful journey. Mindfulness practices such as meditation can help individuals stay grounded and move through the various states of consciousness induced by magic mushrooms. Setting intentions provides a framework for experience.

6.3.6 Personal Health Assessment

Conducting a personal health assessment, including mental health considerations and drug interactions, is essential before embarking on magic mushrooms. Individuals with pre-existing medical conditions or those taking medication should consult a healthcare professional to assess potential risks.

6.3.7 Hydration and nutrition

Staying properly hydrated and nourished is essential to the magic mushroom experience. Staying hydrated and eating light, easily digestible foods contributes to physical well-being and comfort. However, individuals may experience changes in appetite and thirst, so finding a balance is essential.

6.3.8 Integration Procedures

Engaging in post-experience integration practices is a crucial aspect of responsible use. Reflection, journaling, and participation in integration circles

provide individuals with the tools
to process and integrate the
insights gained during the
journey into their daily lives.

6.3.9 Legal Awareness

Understanding the legal status of
magic mushrooms in your locality
is essential for responsible use.
Compliance with the law and the
enforcement of sound drug
policies contribute to a safer and
more informed environment for
individuals interested in
researching these substances.

The Legal Landscape

The legal status of magic mushrooms varies widely across jurisdictions, shaping the landscape for their use, cultivation and distribution. This thesis examines the different legal frameworks governing magic mushrooms in different regions and the ongoing evolution of policies regarding these mushrooms.

7.1 Global variability

The legal status of magic mushrooms is subject to considerable variability worldwide. While some countries have decriminalized or legalized their use for personal use, others maintain strict prohibitions. The legal environment is influenced by cultural attitudes, historical context and evolving perspectives on drug policy.

7.2 Decriminalization and Legalization

In some regions, there has been a move towards decriminalization or even legalization of magic mushrooms. Decriminalization often involves reducing the criminal penalties for keeping personal data and treating it as a civil or administrative offence. Legalization, on the other hand, allows regulated access for personal or medical use.

7.3 Medical and therapeutic use

Growing recognition of the therapeutic potential of magic mushrooms has prompted shifts in legal attitudes. Some jurisdictions allow medical or therapeutic use under controlled and controlled conditions. This includes the administration of psilocybin therapy by trained professionals.

7.4 Research and Clinical Trials

Renewed interest in psychedelics, including magic mushrooms, has led to increased research and clinical trials investigating their therapeutic applications. Regulatory authorities in some countries may grant approval for research purposes, allowing scientists to investigate the safety and effectiveness of these substances.

7.5 Challenges and Defenses

Despite changing perspectives, challenges remain in advancing more progressive drug policies. Stigma, misinformation, and historical prejudice against psychedelics contribute to resistance in changing legal frameworks. Advocacy groups seek to dispel myths, promote evidence-based policy, and highlight the potential benefits of responsible psychedelic use.

7.6 Legal Risks and Consequences

Tampering with magic mushrooms in areas where they are illegal carries legal risks and consequences. Individuals caught in possession, cultivation or distribution may face criminal prosecution, fines or imprisonment. Legal awareness and compliance with local regulations are essential to mitigating these risks.

7.7 Development of legislation

Legislative developments related to mushrooms are dynamic. Some jurisdictions are actively revising and amending existing laws to better reflect current attitudes and scientific knowledge. Monitoring legislative changes is essential for individuals who want to navigate the legal environment responsibly.

7.8 Public Opinion and Policy Making

The public's perception has a big influence on drug policy. Changing societal attitudes toward psychedelics, along with increased awareness of their potential benefits, may influence policymakers to reconsider existing legal frameworks. Public education and dialogue contribute to the promotion of informed perspectives.

Note: This book is for informational purposes only and does not encourage or condone the illegal use of magic mushrooms. It is essential to know the legal status of these substances in your jurisdiction and to approach their use responsibly and safely.

TABLE OF CONTENTS